experiencing
DEMENTIA

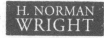

H. NORMAN WRIGHT

PUBLISHING GROUP

NASHVILLE, TENNESSEE

978-1-4336-5023-9

Published by B&H Publishing Group,
Nashville, Tennessee

Dewey Decimal Classification: 616.8
Subject Heading: DEMENTIA \ MENTAL HEALTH \
MEDICAL CARE

1 2 3 4 5 6 7 8 • 21 20 19 18 17

Contents

For God is not the author
of confusion, but of peace.

1 Cor. 14:33 NKJV

In thee, O LORD, do I put my trust:
let me never be put to confusion.

Ps. 71:1 KJV

Introduction

❦

I have lived the life of a caregiver. At the time, I'm
not sure I realized that was my reality. In fact, I
have been responsible for several individuals in this
way.

You may be at a place where it dawns upon you
that you've either become a caregiver or you are facing that prospect in the immediate and ongoing
future.

In my case, my wife and I cared for our pro-
foundly mentally disabled son who was born with
brain damage and an improperly formed brain.
Matthew died at twenty-two.

We also helped care for my mother-in-law for
several years as dementia and Alzheimer's took their
toll.

A few years later my wife Joyce was afflicted with
a brain tumor, and we struggled with it for four years
until it returned, expanded, and then took her life.

As I reflect back over the years of caring for loved ones, in each case it was their brain that was affected. And that is what we are facing in this book—understanding how dementia impacts the brain.

Do you avoid using and dislike hearing the sound of the word *dementia*? When many of us hear it mentioned, we know it's not good news. We would rather avoid it, but what do we really know about it?

We need to know as much as we can about this condition in order to truly understand and help those who suffer from it. It is definitely more than one disease. There are different forms of dementia, like meandering streams branching off from a river. They take different paths as they progress that, if we are not knowledgeable about, can throw us off balance.

The more you know about the different kinds of dementia, the more you can be of help to your family and friends so you're aware in advance of the various needs that will arise, as well as what to expect. The more information you have, the more equipped you'll be to handle the progression of this disease and the changes that will occur. The more you know will diminish the amount of surprises and ambushes you will experience. The phrase, "I wish I knew that," can be lessened and even eliminated if you will follow through with the recommended reading in this introductory book. There will be topics in this book to read and discussions with your loved one you would rather not have to experience, but they are necessary. It's important to talk with your loved one as soon as possible about their care as well as their end-of-life concerns. If you are like most of us, you want the best care for your loved one, so it is important that you stay abreast of the latest research, especially on medications and studies that could improve the remaining life of the person.

CHAPTER 1

You're Not Alone

Your calling to take care of a person with dementia will take more than money and help from other family members. It's a giving of yourself as a person, which includes time, energy, commitment, and love. It also means you will enter a new world of continuous loss as you watch someone you love slip away from you, and there is nothing you can really do to stop the process. You will enter a world of upheaval as you watch this disease continue. Add this to all of your other responsibilities, and you may feel as though you're carrying the weight of the world upon your shoulders. As one daughter said, "I feel like I'm doing it all and there's no relief. Others don't understand!" and they may not. Don't count on receiving thanks or recognition from others. You may end up feeling invisible.[1]

This book has not been easy for me to write. Many thoughts and feelings were activated because I walked this path with my wife, Joyce, for more than two years. I didn't realize how much anticipatory grief I was in until after she died. Part of my knowing that she would die from her brain tumors wasn't always conscious. The surgeries, chemo, and radiation all held out the hope of healing, and our focus was on that; yet under the surface was the entertainment of another possibility—death. Perhaps that stemmed from the death of our son, Matthew, in 1990, after a two-week stay in the hospital for corrective surgery.

One of the greatest gifts we have ever received is our mind—our thoughts and especially our imagination. With it we can be creative and resourceful and move forward in life. But it can also be one of the greatest sources of pain because of what we choose to dwell upon. What we think about and say to ourselves feeds our emotions and our grief. Imagination is to our emotions what illustrations are to a text, or what music is to a ballad. Often we fixate on thoughts and questions that plague the pathways of our mind.

I Wonder . . .

Do you ever wonder what goes through the minds of others? I have. I still do, and especially what went through Joyce's during her last weeks of life. It causes me to wonder what I would think and feel were I in her circumstance and place in life. It causes me to wonder what I *will* think and feel when it is my time to die. At age seventy, and because Joyce is already gone, that is much more real than ever before. I see it less as an ending and more as a transition—a beginning. The hundreds of cards and e-mails I have received in the past month have had a consistent theme that leads to a sense of comfort and reassurance. But every now and then I still wonder.

I wonder . . .

- What went through Joyce's mind each morning when she woke knowing there was a sleeping enemy within her head that could awaken at anytime—and eventually did?

- How much of her thoughts and feelings were for herself or for what this was doing to her loved one? And knowing Joyce as I did, I think I know, since she cared so much for others.

- What she experienced when she asked, "How long?" and heard, "It could be two weeks, or a month, or two." What is it like when you are told the news and then experience the process slowly as symptoms intensify and the words and thoughts diminish?

- What frustration it must have been to think you've said something clearly and then see the puzzlement and wonderment on the faces of others and realize you didn't say what you thought.

- Did the pain and discomfort at the last overshadow looking forward to going to heaven? Could she remember the comfort of the Scriptures? Could she remember and hear and feel our expressions of love? I hope so.

I have a number of other wondrous thoughts. But they will remain in this state, at least for now. "Finally, brothers, whatever is true, whatever is noble, whatever is right, whatever is pure, whatever is lovely, whatever is admirable—if anything is excellent or praiseworthy—think about such things" (Phil. 4:8).

Perhaps you relate to these thoughts and questions that I had. Perhaps they are ones you may want to consider at this time.

If you are reading this book, it is because you either already understand the feelings I am talking about, or you are preparing yourself for what is to come. You may feel like you're on a "never-ending roller coaster" that affects you and everyone else.[2] Take heart! You are not alone.

Allow the information and suggestions in this book to give you a deeper understanding of what your loved one is going through, and a plan on how to best love them through it.

Chapter 2

The World of Dementia

This book is definitely a basic introduction. From here your work begins as you expand your knowledge, understanding, resources, and your support system.

You've heard the term *dementia*. Yes, it's true, it's become one of those words that strikes fear into just about everyone. It's the disease we wish was rare, but sadly is not. It can totally strangle our life when it strikes and creates upheaval with our family.

Dementia—what is it? How do you explain it? The dictionary states it is severe impairment or loss of intellectual capacity and personality integration due to the loss or damage to neurons in the brain. Trying to diagnose this isn't all that easy. There is no real test that gives you a "yes" or "no" answer; so many with this problem don't even understand that they have it since they've lost much of their mental ability.

The changes start out so small they could be ignored. They don't seem that important, but the irritants continue. It's the little personality changes that grow and tell us the message that something is not right. In a sense it may feel like the beginning of the end.

Those with dementia have minds that are hard for you to keep up with. They seem to be able to teleport. They jump from place to place—one minute they're present here, and then they think it's fifteen years earlier. Don't try to correct them—it won't help. A dementia brain has lost its ability to deal with stimuli in the way that you and I do.

Let's remember that lifelong habits do not go away with dementia. They will continue to surface and beg to be satisfied. It is our job as their support to see how we can help this to occur. This may stretch our ability. We will need to sit down and recall those habits, and make a list. It's not a one-time exercise, so have your list out and as they come to mind, write them down. Very often we forget and don't make the connection between our loved one's behavior and old patterns of living life. They are trying to hold on to what they had, and by helping them we can make it easier on everyone.[3]

Dementia affects the brain, and gradually lessens its ability to be as functional mentally as it once was. It impacts how the person acquires, understands, and uses information that they gather through their senses. With the new tests that have been developed, doctors can now look at the brain and actually see the changes.

We know so much more about dementia than was known one or two decades ago. For example:

- It is *not* the natural result of aging.
- It *is* caused by specific, identifiable diseases.
- Diagnosis is vital to identify treatable conditions.
- It is vital to have a thorough evaluation to know how to manage the diseases.

Dementia is not really a disease in itself, but a group of symptoms that result from other sources, or diseases. It does not mean crazy. It's a condition within the brain that reduces the ability to remember, think, reason, and judge. It's a relational condition as it reaches out to control and impact others.

Dementia affects the following:

- Memory
- Executive thinking
- Language and speech
- Behavior and social skills
- Movement
- Visual and spatial perception

Dementia and all its variations are thieves. They slowly steal what a person has worked on obtaining their whole life—memories and abilities. You end up with a gradual form of permanent amnesia because of brain cell deterioration and death.

This results in a different type of suffering—this disease does not bring physical pain in and of itself, but a great deal of emotional pain to the person and to their loved ones.

When the symptoms begin to interfere with everyday life, it's said the person has dementia. As I have said, this is a catch-all word that describes many different symptoms.[4]

CHAPTER 3

The Cause of Dementia

Perhaps one of the most common questions is, "What causes dementia?" Unfortunately, what we know is still not certain, but researchers think there are two processes that occur.

First of all, you and I have what is called plaque lurking in our brain. It's a protein fragment and for most of us our brain clears away those fragments and they don't accumulate that much. But for some of us they do start to accumulate over time. Someone suggested the protein fragments become the villain since they begin to clump together into plaques and start to do their dirty work. As they grow, they begin to damage and then destroy brain cells. They hinder the communication process between cells. But the dirty work doesn't stop there. The plaque affects the spaces between the brain cells, but this isn't the only protein

hard at work in a destructive way. Another one is
called the *tau*. You and I have *tau* in our brain and we
need them. Their job is to keep cellular traffic mov-
ing through the cell so the cell can function. But
when these twist together they're called *tangles* and
slow down and block the transportation of nutri-
ents—which we need in and out of the cells—as well
as begin to destroy neurons. It's as though they begin
to drive fifty, then forty, then thirty miles an hour in
the fast lane of the freeway. What's the result of this
blockage? Brain cells degenerate and subsequently
die. It doesn't just happen to one brain cell but can
damage accompanying cells and spread throughout
the brain. Part of the overall damage is the shrinkage
of the brain.

We don't know whether it's a plaque or a tau that
is the most responsible for the problem of dementia.
They both destroy brain cells and can be at work as
much as ten to twenty years before it becomes out-
wardly obvious.[5]

Let's look into your brain a little deeper, to understand this deadly invader. Plaque and tangles show
up first in the regions of the brain responsible for
memory. They then fulfill their goal of robbing the
brain of other functions as well.[6]

CHAPTER 4

The Brain

Your brain—it only weighs three pounds, regardless of your weight. Without this organ your heart wouldn't beat, your lungs couldn't breathe, and your limbs would be immobilized. This unique mass directs what you do. It's amazing in what it does, but it's also home to your consciousness. It changes every minute of every day. And more than 90 percent of what we know about it has been discovered in the last ten years. It's involved in all you experience in life including your past and present.[7]

Dementia impacts and erodes a section called the hippocampus, a section involved in the forming of memories and their storage. There are many pathways to this emotional center. The hippocampus is larger in women, and yes, women do tend to have better memories especially if emotions are involved.

The more this section is impacted by plaque and tangles the more difficult it is to form new memories and to reach back for older memories!

As the disease moves through the hippocampus, it spreads to other portions of the brain. This creates a growing loss. We experience losses throughout our lives, but one of the most difficult is the loss of yourself. This is what is gradually occurring.

Another part of our brain that is impacted is the amygdala, which is the alarm section of the brain. Sometimes it's referred to as the sentry. If a cat knocks over a vase at night and you hear it and react, this is the section that alerts you. It can hijack other portions of the brain. It's responsible for the creation of emotions and their memories. Many of the emotional issues and personality changes seen in Alzheimer's have their origin here because it's the site and centerpiece of your emotional system.

The portion of the brain stem that is involved in sleep is also affected, which accounts for the sleeplessness that is experienced.[8]

Each region of the brain communicates via an extensive two-way network of neurons. And this affects all the functions of the brain.

If someone asked you, "Why did this occur?" just say, the symptoms of dementia are related to the consequences of having areas of the brain that are no longer functioning.[9]

CHAPTER 5

Memory

The loss of memory is frightening and devastating. How can we think about the present and the future when it is based upon memories and experiences of the past? It is our history, and it's used to help us make sense of our lives. Memory shapes and controls our lives more than we can ever fully grasp. When your memory is impaired, you are no longer you. The writers of Scripture knew the value of remembering.

> "I will remember the covenant between me and you and all living creatures of every kind." (Gen. 9:15)

> Remember, Lord, your great mercy and love, for they are from of old. (Ps. 25:6)

Jesus said, "This is my body given for you; do this in remembrance of me." (Luke 22:19)

When we lose our memories, we lose our history and who we are. Our memories give us life.

IMMEDIATE MEMORY

This is where you remember what was just said in a conversation. But if your short-term memory isn't working, you may not remember that the conversation even occurred.

SHORT-TERM MEMORY

This has a very important function. We use it to remember what has happened today or our plans for today and tomorrow. This memory helps you multi-task, so when it is impacted, the person can only focus on one thing at a time. When short-term memory is affected, usually complex tasks come to a halt such as preparing meals, working, and hobbies.

One of the signs of short-term memory loss is repetitive questioning. It's difficult for a person to remember they've been asking the question again and again, but they will understand when they are being criticized or if you're upset.

WORKING MEMORY

This memory allows you to mentally hold onto information while processing it. With the disease you will be unable to add or subtract, as you will not be able to hold on to the numbers. This type of memory also helps divide our attention.[10]

PROCEDURAL

By doing the same thing over and over again a new long-term memory is established. This would include activities like brushing your teeth or taking out the trash. These are activities that are repeated to the point of becoming "second nature" as some would call it.

If you're like most individuals when dementia is mentioned, what comes to mind is Alzheimer's, but that is only one of the variations. Dementia is basically an umbrella term used to describe many of the symptoms that interfere with our everyday functioning.[11]

Chapter 6

Types of Dementia

Alzheimer's accounts for somewhere between 60 to 80 percent of all cases and is what we will be spending a majority of this book focusing on; but, what are the other types? Let's consider the five most common.

Vascular Dementia

Vascular dementia is thought to be the second or third most common cause of dementia, accounting for 12 to 20 percent of all dementia. It occurs because of a series of small and/or silent strokes, some of which are so small it's difficult to note any changes. Perhaps you have heard of TIAs (Transient Ischemic Attack) or mini strokes. Blood vessels that have been hardened or blocked stop the blood from flowing to parts of your brain. Thus your brain cells in these areas die. Symptoms are similar to Alzheimer's.

DEMENTIA WITH LEWY BODIES

This is another type of dementia, which is difficult to distinguish from Alzheimer's. It occurs because abnormal clumps of protein form in a section of the brain causing nerve cells to degenerate.

You've probably heard of Parkinson's disease. This is caused by the same proteins, but they form deep within the brain causing tremors and problems with movement.

FRONTOTEMPORAL DEMENTIA

This affects the person's personality as well as their behavior since the section of the brain responsible for behavior is gradually eroded. Inappropriate and compulsive behaviors may begin to emerge.

NORMAL PRESSURE HYDROCEPHALUS

This used to be called "water on the brain." It occurs because of the buildup of fluid in the brain. Headaches, dizziness, changes in personality and behavior, as well as memory loss can occur.[12]

MILD COGNITIVE IMPAIRMENT

As you continue to learn about dementia, you will hear about MCI. This stands for mild cognitive impairment. This is technically not a dementia, and only about half of those affected move onto Alzheimer's. The first symptom is a progressive memory loss, but they are still functional and can maintain their own independence. Some who have MCI progress quickly, while others live with this for ten years. "This term is used to identify people who complain of memory difficulties and who are found to have declined modestly on tests of memory. Ten to 12 percent of individuals with this set of symptoms develop dementia in each subsequent year for at least five years."[13]

Remember, Alzheimer's is the most common of the cases and overshadows others in terms of number and severity of the care challenges.

Chapter 7

Alzheimer's

Alzheimer's disease comes silently, like little cat's feet, except that cat's feet are soft, loving and remembering—not harsh, disrupting and destroying. It is such a deceiving, disorienting, "first you see it, now you don't" kind of disease that defining when and where it strikes is almost impossible. It hides its depredations behind behaviors already a part of the patient's personality so that it is in full flower before recognized as the devourer it truly is. It is our task as caregivers to make sure that we define the limits between the disease and the person for whom we care. We must never despise the person, we must always despise and fight the disease.[14]

There are different diseases that can lead to dementia, some of which we discussed in the previous chapter, but Alzheimer's is the most common, accounting for somewhere between 60 and 80 percent of all cases of dementia. There are about 5.3 million people who are stricken by this disease. And that doesn't include all who are impacted by it. Dementia doesn't just change, the person who is afflicted with the disease. It reaches out with an invitation to many others to also change and it's an invitation that cannot be refused. Think of all the family members whose lives are changed as they have to adapt to the changes in their loved ones and thus change their own life.

Why is this number going up? Over the course of the last century a number of factors, such as medical advances, widespread access to health care, improved sanitation, and better nutrition have had a tremendous impact on how long we live. With the Baby Boomer generation on the verge of retirement, we are now looking at a shift to an even older society. This disease usually hits after age sixty-five but can occur as early as thirty.[15]

Why are we seeing an increase in the number of people diagnosed with Alzheimer's? Why do more women than men get Alzheimer's? It's not anything genetic, or environmental. It is simply that we are living longer, and women traditionally live longer than men.[16]

This is a disease that progresses through various stages. If your loved one has been diagnosed as being in stage 1 or 2, they are not yet labeled as having the Alzheimer's disease.

The first stage of the disease can occur without any symptoms. Memory may not be as sharp as it once was, but that could be for a number of reasons. In order to say that a person is headed for this disease, brain imaging would need to be used to show that plaques are being formed.

The second stage shows a number of symptoms, but they are not severe enough to cause loss of independence. This stage is called *Mild Cognitive Impairment* or MCI. In spite of some memory lapses and some confusion, they still function with daily living tasks and on their own. Only about half of those with MCI eventually move to the next stage and develop Alzheimer's. For some the progression is rapid while others it's very slow.

Stage 3 is definitely Alzheimer's. The brain has started to shrink because of the plaques and tangles. All the symptoms are quite apparent and care from others is necessary.

Alzheimer's is overwhelming. Think about this, "Although there are many contenders for world's cruelest disease, Alzheimer's ranks right up there—cunningly and brilliant, turning capable adults into babies, and petulant babies at that. More than any other kind of death, family members of people with Alzheimer's experience massive relief. One woman said, 'I lost my mother twice, once to Alzheimer's, and once to death.'"[17]

CHAPTER 8

Progression of
the Disease

How does it begin and what can you do? Your loved one is not the same. You may even struggle admitting it, but no matter how you try to explain it away, it's Alzheimer's. It may be forgetfulness, confusion, or behavior, and personality changes.

MEMORY

Our memory is actually a collection of several memory systems, some of which we discussed previously. And each one has different purposes. The portion you use for addition and subtraction will be different from when you reflect on a special vacation.

The way the disease manifests itself also varies from person to person. Some live for two to three years while others live for ten to twenty. Sometimes their memory works in one area but not in another. It can be very confusing for those witnessing the changes, but we will look at the most common progression.

When the disease hits, the first memories to be impacted are recently acquired facts and events, or short-term memory, rather than long-term. It's easy to forget appointments and conversations. You may forget recent experiences but remember an event or experience ten to twenty years ago. Acquired skills and procedures may remain intact even longer. And this is not something a person does deliberately or has any choice in. This is the area that is damaged first before it spreads to other areas.

This may cause a person to have constant questions about what is going on and may even repeat the same questions. It may be difficult to hear the same question again and again. You will need an abundance of patience since the best way to respond is to answer the question as though it is the first time it has been asked. This helps prevent the person from feeling humiliated. Some have found it helpful to use white boards or poster board with answers to commonly asked questions or important information.[18]

In the loss of short-term memory, daily events are no longer stored so what *does* the person think about? The memories from the past that are available to them. Thus much of their conversation will be about the past.

This may seem redundant to you. You may be tempted to lose patience with the person. You may expect them to remember. Don't. In your heart and mind give them permission to not remember and you will have an easier time. The phrase, "What do you mean you don't remember? I told you . . ." is *not* helpful. You won't always understand them—what they say or do—and that's all right.

They will misplace things. Just expect this to happen. You may need to repeat statements again and again. A new person may need to reintroduce themselves throughout a conversation.

Here are some other characteristics of short-term memory loss to keep in mind.

They may have difficulty keeping themselves occupied or entertained.

They progressively lose the capacity to distinguish what's relevant and what's not.

If they feel overwhelmed by a family gathering or going to a restaurant, they may want to leave. They can't take into consideration how what they do impacts others.

The reality is that because of what is happening in their brain it's difficult for them to get through a day. It's difficult for them to figure everything out.[19]

> Being thoughtful about the person with short-term memory loss means helping them compensate for that loss in the events of their daily life and being mindful of the emotional changes that accompany this loss. Carers need to approach the person with dementia in a way that helps them to relax, to feel safe and secure. Helping them to stay safe in the use of medication and use of the stove are high priority. Being gracious, when the person with dementia is forgetful, means: answering a repeated question as if it was the first time of asking; refraining from reasoning and arguing; and, neither expecting them to remember, nor becoming upset when they forget.[20]

For example, the taking of medication is impacted by short-term memory. Yes, they may remember, "I took those pills," but not how many. You may need to work with specialists and medical staff to solve this problem.

Keep in mind when the disease is beginning, short-term memory fluctuates from working to not working. This will be frustrating and confusing to both you and your loved one. It will start out being difficult to learn something new, but eventually the short-term memory will shut down completely.

As Alzheimer's progresses, the impairment will move on to the working memory. With an unaffected brain, you can participate in a conversation while remembering that you need to turn off the stove in five minutes. If you have Alzheimer's, you have difficulty dividing your attention, so the oven stays on.

At this point, names and identities of close friends and family can start to get confusing. As memories start to vanish, relationships become fuzzy.

In the most severe stage, procedural memory begins to disappear. There may still be recognition of people or tasks, but the brain is no longer able to understand what to do with that information.[21]

Eventually the long-term memory is impacted. Because of the effect on the short-term memory, it's difficult to have memories make it into long-term. Sometimes this is referred to as a retrograde amnesia. Many seem to have a heightened ability to remember their early years. And what they do remember is not always in the correct sequence.

You've probably put a puzzle together. You're able to piece it together by using other similar pieces to make connections. You look for patterns and color similarities, and eventually all the pieces come together. The disappearance of long-term memory is like taking piece after piece out of the puzzle and discarding it. With Alzheimer's it's difficult to understand and create a complete picture. They may have some individual memories, but they no longer have the connections of how they fit together into one life.[22]

And this can fluctuate—one day they remember very little while another day they are sharp as a tack. Keep in mind that a person with dementia may not be aware that their long-term memory is fading. They are not bothered by the changes, and they trust their memory even though parts may be wrong. Arguing and trying to correct them is counterproductive and will only cause both you and them to become frustrated and hurt.

Emotions also play a large role in what memories are affected by Alzheimer's. For everyone, emotional events or investments are remembered most easily. Strong emotional impact locks events in the memory. You may be surprised at the memories that are easily recalled by someone suffering from later stages of Alzheimer's.[23] (For information on memory loss with other types of dementia different from Alzheimer's, see Jennifer Ghent-Fuller, *Thoughtful Dementia Care,* Amazon CreateSpace, 2012.)

COMMUNICATION

The ability to intelligibly express yourself with language tends to deteriorate faster than the ability to comprehend words and sentences. Many with Alzheimer's have trouble finding the right words to express what they want to say. They understand the conversation, and they know what they want to say but cannot access the words to express it.

Those in the mild stage of Alzheimer's disease are still able to have coherent conversations. They can read out loud, understand what they're reading, and write complete sentences. In the moderate stage, they continue to be able to read and understand what they are reading, and comprehend what people say to them. Unfortunately, the ability to formulate coherent sentences and to name objects diminishes. As it becomes more difficult to retrieve desired words, speech may become vague and imprecise. And as the ability to produce spontaneous sentences diminishes, the person may resort to repeating commonly used phrases over and over in a conversation.

In the last or severe state, language comprehension and expression are both severely diminished. However, a person in the severe stage may still be able to recognize his or her name and respond when addressed directly. The ability to produce coherent sentences will vary from person to person. At this stage, some people with Alzheimer's disease do not speak at all.[24]

One of the issues you will need to confront is the language difficulties that can occur. Aphasia is one that happens gradually as the dementia intensifies. It's the loss of language. Dementia is a thief. It is constantly robbing your loved one. It robs them of their vocabulary and grammar. They struggle understanding what you say or mean and what they once knew; they are now at a loss for words. It's not easy for them to respond to questions. It helps to allow the person permission to interrupt a conversation so they won't forget what they wanted to say.

Sometimes body language is better than words—smiles, gestures, tone of voice, facial expression, stroking, etc., can be helpful. Unfortunately, as time goes on, your loved one may lose all their language function. But don't let that stop you from conversing with them.[25]

As the disease intensifies, so do the symptoms. As language ability deteriorates, they may express agitation through behaviors such as screaming, pacing, and an inability to sit calmly. People in the moderate or later stages of the disease may wander aimlessly from room to room.

Communicating with family members who are unimpaired can be a task in itself, but when any kind of dementia hits, frustration can intensify. Not only does your loved one struggle to find the right words, but you will struggle to adapt your expression so understanding occurs. There is no magic way to communicate except to follow this guideline: keep it simple and direct.

Here are some ways you can help make communication easier:

- Keep all distractions to a minimum such as television, radio, iPhone, iPads, etc., when you are talking to the person.
- Keep your voice low and calm. A lower pitch is easier to hear. Sometimes a gentle touch helps.
- Speak slowly and clearly. Make sure they hear you.
- Use simple sentences that convey only one idea or instruction at a time. They cannot remember too many items. What makes sense to you may be too much for them.
- Whatever you need to say, try to make it positive.
- Avoid using pronouns such as he, she, they, and it. This is too general. Instead, refer to every object or person by name.
- Be patient and allow enough time for the person to hear and think about what you're saying.
- If necessary, repeat statements in the same way several times until you get a response. Be aware that your tone can convey frustration.
- Use gestures or pictures to help get your point across. Do this slowly.[26]

CONFUSION

Insight on the part of your loved one is limited and diminishing. Sometimes they may realize the problem, while other times they may have no idea why thinking has become so difficult. Frustration and anger can emerge. It's difficult to convince someone of something when their own mind is against them. Thinking processes will change since abstract thought becomes progressively difficult for them.

Some are confused about how to respond socially. They may act inappropriately in social situations, using coarse language or telling crude jokes. They enjoy social events but may avoid them because of embarrassment about their condition and their inability to respond appropriately.

Expect disorientation. It will progress from getting lost in new areas, to confusion in familiar neighborhoods, and eventually disorientation in their own home. Your safety concerns will elevate as they become more and more dependent.

What can you expect from the person about time and orientation? Confusion! And this increases with the progression of the disease. This includes dates, days, and time. The more unfamiliar locations in the area the more difficult it is.

In the moderate stage, time orientation worsens. Someone in this stage may think they're living in another period of life. They now have trouble finding their way around even in familiar places. They may not recall where to put items. It's particularly important at this stage for people with Alzheimer's to be supervised and to have identification in case they become lost. The Alzheimer's Association provides the "Safe Return" program.

Don't be surprised at some of the behavioral changes. They may become more irritable than usual or get angry without provocation. Agitation and aggression can develop, even in the mildest person. Those who were very social and outgoing may become subdued or their responses could be intensified.

SENSORY

There is a grouping of changes that make it difficult for you and your loved one—these affect day-to-day functioning. It's the ability to use the senses—vision, hearing, smell, taste, touch, and temperature. Their senses are not working properly.

Losses abound here. This includes the loss of visual depth perception: how close objects are, or the height of chairs, not remembering a curb, and lack of peripheral vision. Smell, taste, hearing are even affected because there is no memory of what the sensation means. What is the ringing of the doorbell, or the clothes dryer, or the smoke alarm? These can be frightening when you do not know what they mean. Even TV can be frightening.

What the senses used to provide as pleasure and soothing may now be experienced as painful and disruptive. Or they may not experience the pain they need to feel and end up with injuries. Their bodies may not send the right messages. When they do feel pain, they may not remember what is causing it or what to do about it.[27]

VISUAL AND SPATIAL

Once again this will intensify as the disease progresses—difficulty with what we think is so simple—visual and spatial. Many people with Alzheimer's disease have problems with visual identification of objects and spatial orientation. A test often used to determine the extent of these problems is called the clock-drawing in which the person draws the face of a clock or copies one.

Visual-spatial impairments make it difficult to perform certain tasks as well as recognize faces and identify objects. They may be unable to recall how common objects, such as a comb, pencil, or hammer, are used. It's the meaning of the object that is lost and not the skills. You will see this problem manifest itself in driving as well.

The extent of disability in this area of ability depends on how much damage has been done to the areas of the brain that control this function.

The ability to solve problems in day-to-day life is troublesome for the person as well as for you if you're the caregiver. For example, a person with Alzheimer's disease may have trouble balancing their checkbook or handling a household emergency. They will also slowly lose the ability to grasp abstract concepts.

In the mild stage of Alzheimer's disease, impairments occur in problem-solving ability and judgment. Some household tasks can be handled, but the ability to handle finances is often the first to deteriorate. The ability to handle finances include managing the checkbook, bill payment, and understanding a bank statement, is already impaired in the mild stage of Alzheimer's disease. This capacity will continue to decline. But in the moderate stage, they are not able to manage money at all.

In the severe stage, problem solving and judgment are quite impaired and even simple decisions must be supervised.

Be aware that verbal or physical aggression may occur when you are helping with everyday things like bathing, grooming, or meal preparation. Remember that some of the frustration you see is from the changes in their life, the ability to understand only some of what is occurring.

OTHER EFFECTS

Loss is the key word with all types of dementia. We've talked about some already, but let's consider some more.

Early in the progression of dementia, they lose their ability to use time. The reminders of time that we experience each day are not in place. They don't work for them as they used to.

Another loss is their initiative. It's difficult for them to start activities or conversations.

Sexual intimacy will probably still continue at first but in time it, too, is lost. This can be a source of confusion and conflict. There are numerous issues about intimacy that need to be addressed. The best material I have found on this is from Jennifer Ghent-Fuller, *Thoughtful Dementia Care*, pp. 100–104.

One issue needs to be explained. It's called *sundowning*—agitation that increases in the evening and nighttime—and is relatively common among people with Alzheimer's. It's not known why this happens, but people with this disturbance experience increased confusion, anxiety, agitation, and disorientation beginning at dusk and continuing through the night. Sundowning may be complicated by sleep disturbances. The person may sleep during the day and stay up all night.[28]

Muscle strength and coordination are affected as seen in handwriting, balance, grasping, walking and duration of movement, and the numerous daily tasks such as shopping, cleaning, repairs. The abilities vary from day to day as well.

And why do all these symptoms occur? The bottom line is simply because certain portions of the brain are not doing what they are supposed to be doing. *They don't work anymore.*

As you have probably realized by now, dementia is a disease that doesn't leave any part of life untouched. It's consuming. And people do die from dementia. They may have other complications, but in and of itself this disease can lead to death since eventually their brain can no longer keep the body breathing. Eventually their heart stops.[29]

CHAPTER 9

Alzheimer's: Let's Review

THE SIGNS

- Memory loss that disrupts daily life including job skills.
- Forgetting recently learned information.
- Forgetting important dates or events.
- Asking for the same information over and over.
- Forgetting names or appointments, but remembering them later.
- Withdrawal from work or social activities or the lack of initiative.

CHALLENGES

- Planning or problem solving.
- Performing familiar tasks, at work or home.

- Changes in ability to develop and follow a plan or work with numbers.
- Trouble following a familiar recipe or keeping track of monthly bills.
- Difficulty concentrating and taking much longer to complete tasks.
- Driving to a familiar location.
- Managing a budget.
- Remembering rules.
- Putting things in inappropriate places.

AREAS OF CONFUSION

- Time or place.
- Seasons and the passage of time.
- Addresses and knowing where they are, how they got there, or how to get back home.
- Understanding an example, or something that happened in the past.
- Misplacing items may cause them to accuse others of stealing.

SENSORY PROBLEMS

- Trouble understanding visual images and spatial relationships and abstract thinking.

- They may forget completely what numbers are and what needs to be done with them.
- Difficulty reading, judging distance, and determining color or contrast.
- Difficulty connecting sounds, smells, and feelings with their meanings.

COMMUNICATION CHALLENGES

- New problems with words, speaking or writing.
- Trouble following or joining conversation.
- They may stop in the middle of a conversation and have no idea how to continue.
- They may repeat themselves.
- They may forget simple words or substitute inappropriate words.

PERSONALITY CHANGES

- They may have trouble keeping up with a favorite sports team or remembering how to complete a favorite hobby.
- They may become extremely confused, suspicious, depressed, or fearful.

- They may be easily upset at home, at work, with friends, or in places where they are out of their comfort zone.
- Their mood swings don't seem to have any reasons.[30]

CHAPTER 10

Where Do You Start?

If there are indications of any type of dementia, don't delay. Find a medical doctor who specializes in these disorders.

Here are ten very important questions to ask the primary care physician for your loved one:

1. What exactly is wrong with my loved one?
2. Can you suggest any resources where I might find out everything there is to know about my loved one's condition?
3. Is this condition treatable?
4. What can I expect or how will the condition progress?
5. What can I do right now as far as caring for my loved one?
6. Do I need any special equipment?
7. Will my loved one have to be on medication?

8. Can you offer the best care for my loved one, or should we seek the help of a specialist?
9. Is this condition hereditary?
10. Is the treatment covered under my loved one's insurance?[31]

If you think that Alzheimer's disease may be the diagnosis, learn as much as you can. Alzheimer's is a progressive, irreversible, neurological disorder. Read everything available to you so that you can ask intelligent questions. Some of the best materials available are listed in this book.

Develop a support group for yourself prior to going for diagnosis. Ask your pastor, church care group, best friends, and so on to join in prayer with and for you, especially on the day scheduled for your physician's visit. Appoint a person to share the results with others so you don't have that burden.

Don't go alone with your loved one to the physician's office. Take along a supportive friend or family member in the event that you are too upset to drive home or deal with your loved one's questions and fears.

Let the family know the diagnosis may be coming. Be sure to include everyone concerned. Don't be surprised at the variety of reactions from friends and family members. There could be a wide range from acceptance to denial.[32]

As a person moves into this disease, you will see them shifting from being independent to dependent. One of your struggles will be to determine what you *should* take over and how much to take over. If you relieve them of some responsibility, remember you're not just taking over a task; you're taking away independence.

You may need to make an evaluation or get a professional evaluation to work out the best progression plan. You will need to decide if your loved one can still do each task completely, safely, and without becoming upset.[33]

Here are some of the most common memory symptoms of Alzheimer's. Some of these may also apply to multiple forms of dementia. Look through these and begin to make notes of which of these you see and how often. Being aware of how severe your loved one's symptoms are will help you to be prepared for the times they will need the most help.

Memory loss that disrupts daily life including job skills. One of the most common signs of Alzheimer's is forgetting recently learned information. Others include forgetting important dates or events; asking for the same information over and over. Sometimes forgetting names or appointments, but remembering them later.

Challenges in planning or solving problems or performing familiar tasks. Some people may experience changes in their ability to develop and follow a plan or work with numbers. They may have trouble following a familiar recipe or keeping track of monthly bills, difficulty concentrating or take much longer to do things than they did before.

Difficulty completing familiar tasks at home, at work, or at leisure. They find it hard to complete daily tasks. Sometimes people may have trouble driving to a familiar location, managing a budget, or remembering rules.

Confusion with time or place. People with Alzheimer's can lose track of dates, seasons, and the passage of time. They may have trouble understanding something if it is not happening immediately. Sometimes they may forget where they are or how they got there.

Trouble understanding visual images and spatial relationships or abstract thinking. They may have difficulty reading, judging distance, and determining color or contrast.

New problems with words in speaking or writing. People with Alzheimer's may have trouble following or joining a conversation. They may stop in the middle of a conversation and have no idea how to continue or they may repeat themselves.

Misplacing things and losing the ability to retrace steps. A person with Alzheimer's disease may put things in inappropriate places. They may lose things and be unable to go back over their steps to find them again. Sometimes they may accuse others of stealing.

Decreased or poor judgment. People with Alzheimer's may experience changes in judgment or decision-making such as the way they handle money or grooming.

Withdrawal from work or social activities or lack of initiative. People with Alzheimer's may start to remove themselves from hobbies, social activities, work projects, or sports. They may have trouble keeping up with a favorite sports team or remembering how to complete a favorite hobby. They may also avoid being social because of the changes they have experienced.

They may be easily upset at home, at work, with friends, or in places where they are out of their comfort zone. They have mood swings that don't seem to have any reason.[34]

Chapter 11

Responding to Alzheimer's

Now that we have looked at the disease, and its effects on an individual, let's get very basic on how you as a loved one can be prepared. We need to learn from the experience of others. Just remember your abilities will be taxed to the extreme. Perhaps some of these suggestions are basic, but it is better to be overly prepared than be told too late and say, "I never thought of that."

How to Prepare

Look at your home the way you would if a toddler was coming for a visit. Make it as safe and comfortable as possible so you don't have to hover and watch your loved one 24/7. You will need to evaluate your current safety measures not just once, but every few months since the person you're caring for can change so frequently.[35] Consider installing devices both in and outside the home that will help to keep your loved one safe and secure.[36]

Help your loved one maintain their self-esteem and independence as long as possible. It helps to focus on what they *can* do rather than what they *cannot* do. But whenever you see they are at any kind of risk to themselves, you will need to become more involved. Safety of the person and those around them is a main consideration.

A person's memory and judgment may be impaired, but they still have feelings. The person may be more or less emotional than in years before. They can sense when you are upset or impatient or frustrated or angry. Like all of us they respond best to love and acceptance. They need the opportunity to express what they are feeling.[37]

Follow these steps when addressing a problem.

Restrict—try to get the person to stop mistakes they are doing.

Reassess—could something else be causing this problem? Would a different approach work?

Reconsider—we always need to consider how things must seem from their point of view.

Re-channel—is there any way that this behavior could continue in a safe environment? What's another option?

Reassure—take the time to give emotional support that things will work out and above all that you care for them.[38]

There are many areas in which a person is going to need changing levels of assistance. Here are just a few:

DRIVING

This is often a problem even after being diagnosed; many don't grasp the need to stop driving. You will need to make the decision—is it safe or not? To take the burden and pressure off of you, ask your doctor to write a "no longer able to drive" letter. You may need to enlist the assistance of the DMV to restrict their driving. Regardless of how you do this, it is often a difficult transition for the person to give up their sense of freedom and independence.

MEDICATION

A person with the disease will need the assistance of someone else to take the right dosage at the right time. They cannot be trusted to take medication correctly. They may not be able to express their need for more or less meds.

FINANCIAL AND LEGAL MATTERS

This is another area where the need for assistance is great but may be resisted. It's more than turning over these items, but it's giving up independence and freedom. It's important to remember this all the way through creating a new world and environment for the person. As long as they are mentally competent, include them in all areas of decisions that are legal, financial, or healthcare related. At some point in time, the control in this area will have to be given to someone else who will act in their best interest.

DIET

Everyone needs a healthy balanced diet. Too often the person has other physical problems, and this along with memory and judgment problems create health and safety risks and even more so if they prepare their own food. Think about all the problems that can occur. Burns, falls, improper preparation, food poisoning, poor appetite, or forgetting to eat altogether.

If you are caring for this person, it is your responsibility to ensure they eat a balanced diet. You can prepare their meals or designate another dependable person to prepare them, or arrange to have meals delivered to the home. You need to make sure they actually eat. You may be able to do this by simple observation, but you may also want to weigh the person on a regular basis to watch for any weight loss. Those with Alzheimer's disease frequently lose weight at this stage because they simply forget to eat.[39]

HEALTHCARE

Since the person usually doesn't care for themselves, you will need to oversee their healthcare. This includes not just medical but the dentist, eyeglasses, and hearing. Often they cannot answer questions, and you will need to be prepared in all these areas.

SOCIAL INTERACTION

There are many social adjustments to consider. At some stages a person may be able to respond in an appropriate manner, and other stages may not. Some try too hard to compensate for all the changes, whereas others may prefer to withdraw, which can lead to depression. Recreational activities need to be safe as well as enjoyable for the person.

Caring for this person will stretch your abilities like never before. The following are just some of what you need to be aware of as you care for this person. You may find some thoughts and suggestions repeated. That's all right since this will be a part of your life from now on.

- They may not be able to take responsibility for their own safety.
- Slight mishaps can be a sign of impending accidents.
- Know what the person can and cannot do, and don't take their word for it.
- Have an emergency plan printed out for every family member.
- Remember the most dangerous room in the house is usually the bathroom. Falls, twists, poisons, burns are just some of what can occur.

CHAPTER 12

Caring for Your Loved One

Caring for a person with dementia takes knowledge about the disease and the person, as well as sensitivity to their world.

If you are caring for a person, you will need flexibility since your loved one has damage spreading throughout their entire brain. Your loved one will eventually lose the functions of everyday life. This is not an easy thing to accept. You will have to pray for strength daily, as well as the ability to accept what is coming.

Your loved one will experience some major losses that will increase their dependence on you. This could include the ability to feed oneself, bathing, grooming, using the toilet, getting dressed, and many others.[40] These can be awkward and embarrassing, for both of you, but when you are caring for them through love there is nothing to be embarrassed about.

A person with dementia is very sensitive to stimuli from their environment and especially sounds. It's easy for us to deal with all large amounts of input and sounds, but for someone with dementia, too much input creates stress and anxiety.

Overstimulation might create overload. High levels of sensory stimulation create stress that the dementia brain is unable to process. Here are some examples of what might create overload:

- Bright lights
- Sounds (too loud, dissonant, or too many at once)
- Too much clutter
- Too many people
- Comings and goings
- Several senses stimulated at once
- Too many choices
- Not enough personal space
- Unwanted touch

On the other hand, not enough sensory stimulation can be just as damaging to the person. Sensory deprivation can happen in a number of ways:

- Not seeing familiar objects or people
- Lack of caring touch
- Food that is bland or not to the person's taste
- Sameness in the days
- Lack of access to nature
- Not having a pet
- Lack of exposure to favorite music
- Monotone surroundings. Being in a foreign environment
- Lack of pleasant smells[41]

When there is an imbalance, you could expect the person to avoid the stimuli or look for stimuli or begin reacting and venting emotionally.

Who is responsible for the right kind of input? You will be. Not too much, but just enough and the right kind. This can only be accomplished through a process of trial and error. You will need to listen and watch.

All this means is you need to be aware of the emotional stimuli they are getting or not getting and make adjustments for them. Much of life is centered around food. It's a source of sensory as well as an important time to interact with others. It will be up to you to get it "right."[42]

One of the unique features of this disease is wandering. It's a pressure for you since the possibility is scary and is always a possibility. It's a danger for your loved one. It could happen at home or at an outing. The environment where it happens could be familiar or new. It's a pressure no matter where you are.

At home you can use locks and alarms. The problem is what works for one person may not work for another. You will need to evaluate exits, and not just conventional exits. It may become necessary to install locks on windows, garage doors, sliding glass doors, and any other openings. It is important to make sure that the living environment is prepared early. Alzheimer's affects every person so differently that you never know how fast a person will progress, or if they will move back and forth between needing and not needing these precautions. It is far better to have a safe place already prepared before it is needed.[43]

Because Alzheimer's is such a growing problem, you will receive suggestions, books to read, websites to browse, and probably end up being overwhelmed by too many suggestions. Your temptation is to try them all. You and your loved one will be frustrated and ready to give up, but don't lose heart! You will find the system that works best for you, and don't worry if it looks different from any of the suggestions you have been given.

Watch out for your expectations. You can't be everything to the person. You're also living on a learning curve. There is so much you don't and won't know at the onset of the disease. You will struggle with the best way to respond. Remorse and guilt may intensify as you struggle with how to best respond to your family member.

You can't control how the disease progresses, nor can you change when and where they will die. Every person will go down a different path with different moods, behaviors, and time frames. I know people who want the disease to progress quickly and others who want to keep their loved one alive, whether they know who they are or not. Unfortunately, neither desire is within our control.

You *can* decide how to look at what is occurring in your life, as well as theirs. Rather than focus on the problems and what is wrong, make a list of your blessings. This is not denial, but recognizing that life is a mixture of joy and sorrow.

Hold their hand. Hug them a lot.

Talk to them—you don't have to know what they can and can't understand. Give them a lot of attention. They may grasp some and not the rest. That is dementia.[44]

Remind yourself that there is so much you don't know and you are not expected to know since all of this is new. You will have to learn new information about this disease. Accept that changes will occur from day to day. Develop your adaptability skills. Accept and expect constant change.

Don't be hard on yourself when you think you've made a mistake. Learn from every interaction. Some practical steps are: apologizing to the person, forgive yourself, listen to your tone of voice, and take an hour break for yourself each day.

Learn as much as possible about the disease and remember that each person will be unique in how they respond and what works for one may not for you.

Don't scold or argue. It won't work. It will put a distance between you and them.[45]

One piece of advice that can be incredibly helpful is: "Jump into reality." Join their world. It won't hurt either of you.[46]

There are certain Scriptures that may help you during this time. This is a time of both fear and confusion for you and for your loved one. In John we read, "Let not your heart be troubled, neither let it be afraid" (14:27 KJV). *Heart* literally means "mind" here and the word *troubled* is a word that means "stirred or agitated." This is often what you feel when you hear the diagnosis—dementia. Don't let what is happening to your loved one force you into fear!

Another verse that can give you stability and even be a source of comfort is 2 Timothy 1:7 (NKJV). "For God has not given us a spirit of fear, but of power and of love and of a sound mind." It's easy to live with fear as your companion as you watch your loved one deteriorate. We talk about confusion as one of the characteristics of dementia. But it's also a tendency for caregivers to experience this as well. Confusion means the loss of orientation, which is the ability to place oneself correctly in the world by time, location, and personal identity. You can easily become overwhelmed by this disease. Scripture addresses this issue of confusion, "For God is not the author of confusion but of peace . . ." (1 Cor. 14:33 NKJV). The more we trust, the less we are confused. "In thee, O LORD, do I put my trust: let me never be put to confusion" (Ps. 71:1 KJV). It comes back to trust. "You will keep in perfect peace those whose minds are steadfast, because they trust in you. Trust in the LORD forever, for the LORD, the LORD himself, is the Rock eternal," (Isa. 26:3–4). "Fear of man will prove to be a snare, but whoever trusts in the LORD is kept safe," (Prov. 29:25). Turn to God as soon as possible. Put your trust in Him, and only there will you find peace.

Part of the purpose of this book is to help you understand what your loved one is going through and to give you suggestions and helps from others who have walked this path before. The final and most important suggestion is to rely on the Word of God and His promises. You will need them.

> For the Spirit God gave us does not make us timid, but gives us power, love and self-discipline. (2 Tim. 1:7)

A Different Type of Grief: Anticipatory

—❧—

O ne wife said, "When all that remained was hope for my husband's survival, and he continued to decline, I felt absolutely helpless. My arsenal was depleted. There was nothing to do but surrender and redefine hope to be much greater than whether he lived or died. In the end, the effort 'to forestall' seemed to cause everyone involved suffering. At the same time, it was an integral part of the journey."

Anticipatory grief is not just focused upon a future loss. It's much more than that. As we work with those in this situation, it's important to be aware of the losses and help the mourner become aware of them. Remember this: the grief that a person experiences during the terminal illness of a loved one is actually stimulated by losses of the past, those that are occurring at the present time, as well as those that are in the future. It's not unusual to remember what they used to experience and to grieve over all that has been taken away that they will never experience again. This is true with dementia.

The loss that you face with a family member with any type of dementia is difficult to handle and grieve over for a number of reasons.

- This loss is confusing, and it is very difficult to make sense of the loss experience (as when a person is physically present but emotionally unavailable).

- Because the situation is indeterminate, the experience may feel like a loss but not be readily identified as one. Hope can be raised and destroyed so many times that individuals may become physically numb and unable to react.

- Because of ongoing confusion about the loss, there are frequent conflicting thoughts and emotions, such as dread and then relief, hope and hopelessness, wanting to take action and then profound reactions and unable to move forward in their lives.

- Because of the ambiguity, and uncertainty, people tend to withdraw instead of offer support because they do not know how to respond, or there is some social stigma attached to the experience.

- Because the loss is ongoing in nature and progressive, the relentless uncertainty causes exhaustion in the family members and burnout of supports.

Sometimes family members begin pulling away from the dying person too soon and engage in premature detachment. They withdraw their emotional investment in the person prior to their death. Many do this in the early stages of dementia. Somewhere I read this statement that impacted my thinking and has stayed with me: "When we interact with a terminally ill person, are we responding to them as if they are dying or as if they are still living?" It's something to consider.

With anticipatory grief, there are three factors impacting your grief: (1) what occurs within you; (2) what occurs between you and your dying loved one; (3) what occurs between you and your family and friends. Let's consider what may be going on within as you await the death.

There are four steps you go through and they overlap. The first one is *growing awareness and acceptance* to the loved one's dying. As time goes on you realize that the illness is much more serious than you thought, and the possibility of their not recovering begins to grow in your mind. Some accept this immediately while others resist it.

You will begin to rehearse the death and its impact and consequences. Then you begin to move into your role as an anticipatory griever.

Your next step is *processing their death emotionally*. This is where a juggling act begins since you are dealing with a multitude of your own emotional reactions to the pending death while having to deal with demands of the other's terminal condition. This is an emotional process that can be quite intense. As if this loss weren't enough, there will be mourning over past losses as well as present and future losses related to this illness.

You come to the place where the reality of their disease and death is so real that you begin to withdraw emotional energy from your loved one as well as all future hopes and dreams.

There are processes or thoughts that go on in your mind as you await someone to die. Thoughts seem to get stuck, and sometimes it seems as if you can't stop thinking about them. There's a gradual transition in your identity, roles, beliefs, and expectations as you begin preparations for the new life without your loved one. All this is occurring while you watch the dementia destroying your loved one. This is the third step.

CONSIDERING THE FUTURE

Your final step is *planning for the future*. It's difficult for some to think about the future without their loved one and what it will be like, but it's necessary to plan. This also involves considering the losses occurring now and what will occur in the future. There will be many decisions to make, but the more equipped you become now, the easier it will be to make the hard choices when the time comes. Keep learning, spend time with your loved one, and rely on God to see you through.

Notes

1. Alexis Abramson, *The Caregiver's Survival Handbook* (New York: A Perigree Book, 2004), adapted, 3.

2. Pauline Boss, *Loving Someone Who Has Dementia* (San Francisco, CA: Jossey-Bass, 2011), adapted, 16–17.

3. Marguerite Manteau-Rao, LCSW, *Caring for a Loved One with Dementia* (Oakland, CA: New Harbinger, 2016), adapted, 38.

4. Kenneth Kosik, *Outsmarting Alzheimer's: What You Can Do to Reduce Your Risk* (Garden City, NY: Reader's Digest, 2015), adapted, 3–4.

5. Ibid., adapted, 4–6.

6. Abramson, *The Caregiver's Survival Handbook*, adapted, 12–13.

7. *The Brain: The Ultimate Guide* (New York: Harris Publishing, 2015), adapted, 7, 27.

8. Kosik, *Outsmarting Alzheimer's*, adapted, 5–7.

9. Jennifer Ghent-Fuller, *Thoughtful Dementia Care* (Seattle, WA: Amazon CreateSpace, 2012), adapted, 4.

10. *2016 Special Report*, "Alzheimer's Disease," adapted, 45.

11. Kosik, *Outsmarting Alzheimer's*, 4.

12. Ibid., adapted, 3–4.

13. Nancy L. Mace and Peter V. Rabins, *The 36-Hour Day: A Family Guide to Caring for People Who Have*

Alzheimer's Disease, Related Dementias, and Memory Loss (New York: Grand Central Life and Style, 2012), 78–79.

14. Elizabeth Hall, *Caring for a Loved One with Alzheimer's Disease* (New York: The Haworth Pastoral Press, 2000), 1.

15. *Healthy Aging*, adapted, 11.

16. Dr. Lorne S. Label, "Dementia Facts and Statistics: Present and Future Published" at: https://www.isnare.com /?aid=282530&ca=Aging.

17. Jennifer Elison and Chris McGonigle, *Liberating Losses: When Death Brings Relief* (Jackson, TN: Da Capo Press, 2004), 53.

18. Ghent-Fuller, *Thoughtful Dementia Care*, adapted, 15–16.

19. Ibid., adapted, 15–28.

20. Ibid., 29.

21. *2016 Special Report*, "Alzheimer's Disease," 45.

22. Ghent-Fuller, *Thoughtful Dementia Care*, adapted, 36–37.

23. See www.disabled-world.com/health/aging/ dementia/statistics.php, 2009.

24. *2016 Special Report*, "Alzheimer's Disease," adapted, 45-46.

25. Merton P. Strommen, *Five Cries of Grief* (Minneapolis, MN: Augsburg Press, 1996), 31.

26. *American Medical Association Guide to Home Caregiving* (Hoboken, NJ: Wiley & Sons, 2001), adapted, 147.

27. Susan Zonnebelt-Smeenge and Robert C. De Vries, *Traveling through Grief* (Grand Rapids, MI: Baker Publishing Group, 2006), 26–27.

28. *2016 Special Report*, "Alzheimer's Disease," adapted, 46-48.

29. Ghent-Fuller, *Thoughtful Dementia Care*, adapted, 160.

30. Ibid., adapted, 4.

31. Gary Barg, *The Fearless Caregiver: How to Get the Best Care for Your Loved One and Still Have a Life of Your Own* (Sterling, VA: Capitol Books, 2001), 128.

32. Hall, *Caring for a Loved One with Alzheimer's Disease*, adapted, 9.

33. Mace and Rabins, *The 36-Hour Day*, adapted, 81.

34. "Alzheimer's Disease," *The Alzheimer's Association*, adapted, 39.

35. Tara Reed, *What to Do Between the Tears* (Portland, OR: Pivot to Happiness, 2015), adapted, 55.

36. Mace and Rabins, *The 36-Hour Day*, 239.

37. National Institute on Aging, *Caring for a Person Who Has Alzheimer's Disease* (Seattle, WA: Amazon CreateSpace, 2013), adapted, 19–26.

38. Mace and Rabins, *The 36-Hour Day*, adapted, 216–17.

39. National Institute on Aging, *Caring for a Person Who Has Alzheimer's Disease*, adapted, 145.

40. Ghent-Fuller, *Thoughtful Dementia Care*, adapted, 182–88.

41. Marguerite Manteau-Rao, LCSW, *Caring for a Loved One with Dementia* (Oakland, CA: New Harbinger, 2016), 72–73.

42. Ibid., adapted, 83.

43. Barg, *The Fearless Caregiver*, 93.

44. Reed, *What to Do Between the Tears*, adapted, 101.

45. Ghent-Fuller, *Thoughtful Dementia Care*, adapted, 18–19.

46. Reed, *What to Do Between the Tears*, adapted, 4.

ADDITIONAL RESOURCES

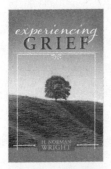

At one time or another, we will all find ourselves facing a dark journey—the passage through grief. *Experiencing Grief* is written for a person who is in the wake of despair grief leaves.

ISBN: 9780805430929

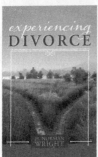

No matter the details, divorce is not a one cut injury. It is a dark journey that a person travels—but does not have to travel alone. *Experiencing Divorce* is written for the person who is in the wake of despair divorce leaves.

ISBN: 9781433650253

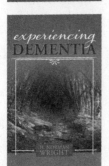

How do you grieve for someone who is still physically with you? *Experiencing Dementia* is written for the person who is in the wake of despair that the diagnosis of Dementia brings.

ISBN: 9781433650239